The
New Mom Thoughts
Keepsake Journal

REAL Questions for Moms with REAL Feelings

By: Ashley D. Shepard

Make this motherhood journey even easier by visiting www.ChefAshleyShep.com/newmom or scanning the QR code on your smartphone's camera to get bonuses that will help you survive the newborn phase and get dinner done faster so you can spend more time with your little one or have a moment to yourself.

New Mom Thoughts

Dedication

I dedicate this book to William, who made me a mother. Though the journey to bring you into the world wasn't easy, it was worth it. I'd do it again in a heartbeat. You are the light to others that I prayed for every day. Also, to your father and my husband, Marshall, thank you for standing by my side every step of the way with loving support.

-Ashley D. Shepard

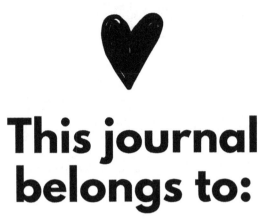

This journal belongs to:

_____

Introduction

I wrote this journal to help new moms explore their thoughts and feelings during their baby's first year. I wish I had something like this during my first few weeks and months with my newborn. This is a safe space to store all the thoughts that cross your mind when worry, lack of sleep, and unmet expectations are all swirling in your head. Whether you feel like you're doing this whole mom thing wrong or you're the perfect example of motherhood, this journal is for you. Processing those thoughts or at least getting them out of your head helps you enjoy the mommy experience and celebrate this new adventure. This journal helps capture all of your new mom feelings during this messy, crazy, and exciting time. Some days are perfectly blissful, while others are filled with constant chaos. Either way, embrace your new normal.

How To Use This Book

Right now, everything in your world is about the baby. But, this book is all about you! It's a place for your highs, lows, best memories, and everything in between. Self-care isn't selfish! When you take care of yourself, it's easier to take care of your baby. Use this journal once a week to explore your thoughts about being a new mom. Since you're probably sleep-deprived (and will be for years to come), you might miss a week - and that's totally fine. Or, maybe you'd prefer to do it more often to get all those thoughts out of your head. It's up to you. There are extra sheets in the back to add more thoughts. Whichever you decide, spend 5-10 minutes journaling each week to check in with yourself. You'll be glad you did. Remember, this is a judgment-free zone. It's just you and your thoughts...no matter how scary or real they may be. There's no right or wrong answer to these questions. Motherhood has its challenges right from the start. However, it's worth it, and so are you.

How I Became a Mother

My pregnancy was pretty easy, but I couldn't say the same for those first few days and weeks after my little one got here. Three days past my due date and many prayers against needing to be induced, my water finally broke. Each labor for my mom was 4 hours or less for her 3 pregnancies. So, as I walked into the hospital that morning, I thought, "We'll have this baby out by lunchtime!" (I was definitely wrong about that.)

Seven hours later, with increasingly stronger contractions, the nurse told me I was 8 cm dilated. Joy began to build as I thought about how soon I would get to meet my son. Though we were "behind schedule," I was still making progress, so that was ok with me. You see, I'm the type of person that likes to plan things out as much as possible to have a clear vision of how they'll go. Meaning, I had already worked out every possible scenario in my head before getting to the hospital. I researched all the things that could go wrong or how my labor would progress. Therefore, I still felt like I was in control of the situation so to speak—as crazy as that sounds. Since this was one of the possible scenarios, I was still at ease with things taking a little longer. It seemed like the time was coming close, so I went ahead and got an epidural.

Hours passed and by dinner time, my doctor arrived to check in on my progress. She informed me that I actually wasn't 8 centimeters...but only 4 or 5. My heart sank a little, but I still remained hopeful that things would progress normally to avoid a c-section. From what I had heard, that recovery was worse than vaginal births. A coworker even told me she wouldn't wish it on her worst enemy. So, clearly, that was definitely not in my plans. Disappointed, but pain-free thanks to my good friend the epidural, I waited patiently to let my body do its thing.

Hours later after trying multiple techniques and pitocin...still no progress. After forty weeks, three days of pregnancy, and 12 hours of labor my fear became my reality: an unplanned c-section. In the moment, I had to accept that the desired option was the safest. This wasn't part of "my plan." Yes, I knew there were a bazillion other things that could have gone wrong but didn't. For that I was 100% grateful. However, it didn't make me any less upset about what was to come. I was upset at the nurse for measuring incorrectly and upset at my body for not doing what it was "made to do." As a woman, that hurt.

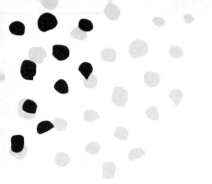

After wiping away my hormone-induced tears, I got myself together, and we prepped for surgery. Thirty minutes later, this beautiful little being who I spent the past 9 months praying over, talking to, and thinking about was finally here! All the worries and stressful thoughts left in an instant. Motherhood became real. My first couple of months postpartum weren't hard because of a colicky baby or complications. Instead, they were harder because my vision didn't match up to my new mom reality. We were blessed with the most perfect baby who only cried when he needed something which was truly a gift. However, I placed a lot of unneeded pressure on myself to "master" this whole motherhood thing when in actuality, I was doing just fine. It was almost as if I needed someone to tell me that everything I was doing was what was best for the baby. (I'm sure those around me told me this exact thing too, but there's a good chance I didn't listen.) Trouble nursing, low milk supply, guilt over supplementing with formula, feeling the need to bounce back from major abdominal surgery, caring for a newborn, and lack of sleep all made me feel extremely overwhelmed. I felt like I just wasn't "good enough". This of course was a lie, but I had a hard time seeing past the pain from surgery and trouble breastfeeding.

As somewhat of a perfectionist, the stress really got to me. I felt like my body didn't do its job during labor and like I was less of a woman because of it. Then after birth, it was failing me yet again by being in the worst pain of my life instead of allowing me to properly care for my newborn. In actuality, my body hadn't betrayed me. It just needed time to heal and rest, but that's not what my head was telling me. It took talking to other moms, lots of time, lots of prayer, lots of tears, and lots of journaling for me to realize this. I finally saw that the "perfect plan" went out the window long ago. Things not going how I thought wasn't my fault. It was also out of my control. What I could control was how I responded to these situations.

It didn't matter that I had to have a c section or that breastfeeding just didn't work out (no matter how hard I tried). All that mattered was that my baby was happy and healthy. And I needed to get back to the same thing for myself and for him. Once I did, I was able to enjoy this new motherhood journey a lot more easily. I had to learn to be gentle with myself...and you need to do the same too momma.

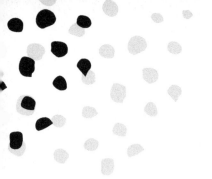

Even if you have a wonderful support system like I did, sometimes, your postpartum brain can work against you. I'm here to tell you to give yourself a break in this thing called motherhood. Your baby being happy and healthy is important, but so is your health and happiness as well. Be patient and know it's a process to learn your baby and figure who you are as a mommy. This journal is here to help you with the process. It's ok to not be okay. But, it's not okay to stay that way.

Was this the hardest thing I've ever done? Yes.
Would I do it again? Absolutely.

I hope this journal helps you to think through your thoughts and feelings, so you can look back on this time and realize just how strong you were and still are.

Signed,
A. D. Shepard

If you or someone you know is suffering from postpartum depression or baby blues, there's help available. It's totally normal to experience this, but know you don't have to go through it alone. Call 1.800.944.4773 or text 503-894-9453 for more information. You can also visit https://www.postpartum.net/ to find out more information about Postpartum Support International. Lastly, flip to the Mommy Resources page at the end of this book for more options.

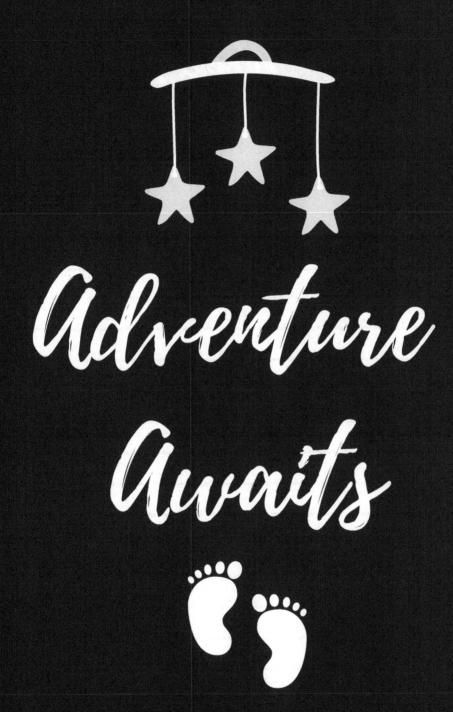

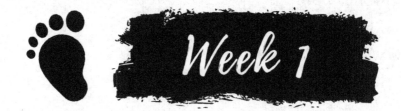

Week 1

What were your first thoughts when you met your baby?

_____
_____
_____
_____
_____
_____
_____
_____
_____
_____
_____
_____
_____
_____
_____
_____

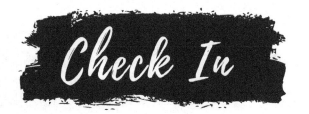

Check In

How are you feeling?
(Ex. happy/sad, worried/hopeful, etc.)

_____

_____

_____

_____

_____

_____

_____

_____

_____

_____

_____

_____

_____

_____

_____

_____

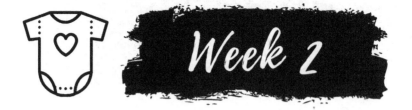

Week 2

Is being a new mom how you thought it would be? Why or why not?

_____

_____

_____

_____

_____

_____

_____

_____

_____

_____

_____

_____

_____

_____

_____

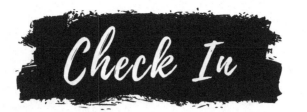

Check In

How are you feeling?

_____

_____

_____

_____

_____

_____

_____

_____

_____

_____

_____

_____

_____

_____

_____

_____

_____

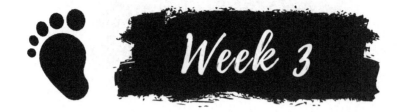

Week 3

What was the first day at home like with the baby?

_____

_____

_____

_____

_____

_____

_____

_____

_____

_____

_____

_____

_____

_____

_____

_____

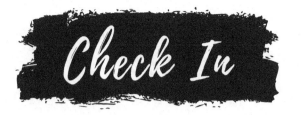

Check In

How are you feeling?

_____

_____

_____

_____

_____

_____

_____

_____

_____

_____

_____

_____

_____

_____

_____

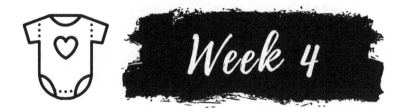

Week 4

What is one thing you wish you would have brought to the hospital/birthing site with you? Why?

_____

_____

_____

_____

_____

_____

_____

_____

_____

_____

_____

_____

_____

_____

_____

_____

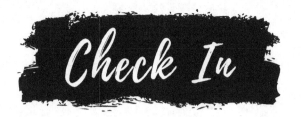

Check In

How are you feeling?

Need help? Check out the New Mommy Resources page
in the back of the book.

_____

_____

_____

_____

_____

_____

_____

_____

_____

_____

_____

_____

_____

_____

_____

_____

Give yourself some

GRACE

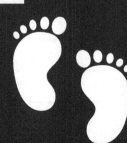

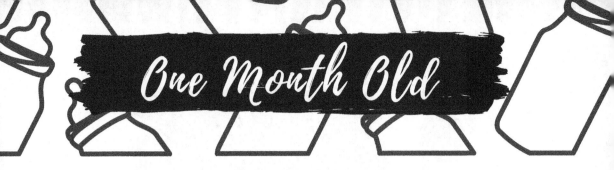

One Month Old

My Baby's Stats
(Height, Weight, Percentiles, etc.)

_____

_____

New Things My Baby Can Do

_____

_____

Things My Baby Likes

_____

_____

Things My Baby Does NOT Like

_____

_____

Favorite memory or mommy accomplishment this month

_____

_____

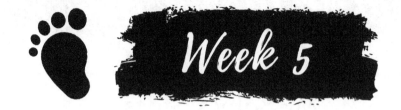

Week 5

What advice would you give to a
fellow mom of a newborn?

_____
_____
_____
_____
_____
_____
_____
_____
_____
_____
_____
_____
_____
_____
_____
_____
_____

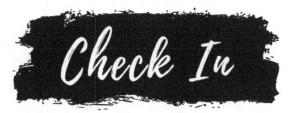

Check In

How are you feeling?
(Ex. happy/sad, worried/hopeful, etc.)

_____

_____

_____

_____

_____

_____

_____

_____

_____

_____

_____

_____

_____

_____

_____

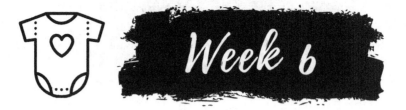

Week 6

What's one thing you can do for yourself today?

_____
_____
_____
_____
_____
_____
_____
_____
_____
_____
_____
_____
_____
_____
_____
_____

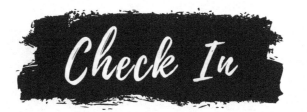

Check In

How are you feeling?

_____
_____
_____
_____
_____
_____
_____
_____
_____
_____
_____
_____
_____
_____
_____

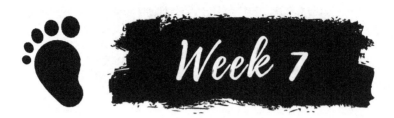

Week 7

Who has been your biggest supporter during pregnancy and/or the first couple weeks with the baby? How?

_____

_____

_____

_____

_____

_____

_____

_____

_____

_____

_____

_____

_____

_____

_____

_____

_____

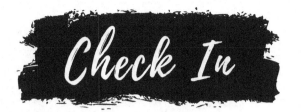

Check In

How are you feeling?

_____
_____
_____
_____
_____
_____
_____
_____
_____
_____
_____
_____
_____
_____
_____
_____

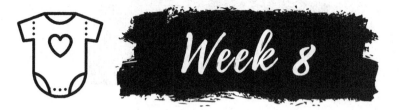

Week 8

Congratulations, you made it two months with your new little one. What's one thing that you've learned about your baby so far?

_____

_____

_____

_____

_____

_____

_____

_____

_____

_____

_____

_____

_____

_____

_____

_____

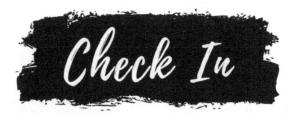

Check In

How are you feeling?

_____

_____

_____

_____

_____

_____

_____

_____

_____

_____

_____

_____

_____

_____

_____

_____

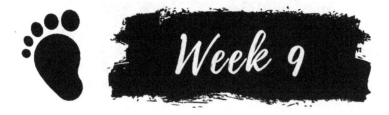

Week 9

What was the best part of your day? The worst part?

_____

_____

_____

_____

_____

_____

_____

_____

_____

_____

_____

_____

_____

_____

_____

_____

_____

_____

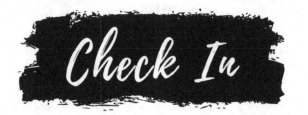

Check In

How are you feeling?

Need help? Check out the New Mommy Resources page
in the back of the book.

_____

_____

_____

_____

_____

_____

_____

_____

_____

_____

_____

_____

_____

_____

_____

_____

_____

Take it
ONE DAY
at a time

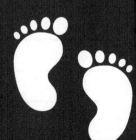

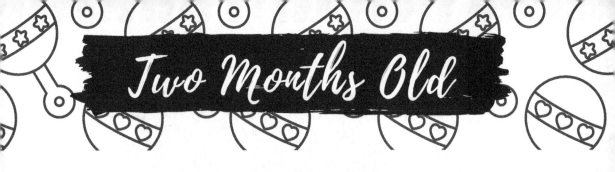

Two Months Old

My Baby's Stats
(Height, Weight, Percentiles, etc.)

_____

_____

_____

New Things My Baby Can Do

_____

_____

_____

Things My Baby Likes

_____

_____

Things My Baby Does NOT Like

_____

_____

Favorite memory or mommy accomplishment this month

_____

_____

_____

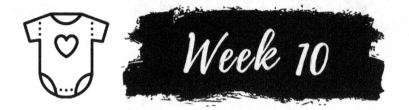

Week 10

Write a letter to your little one to read when they're older.

_____
_____
_____
_____
_____
_____
_____
_____
_____
_____
_____
_____
_____
_____
_____
_____
_____
_____

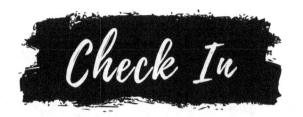

Check In

How are you feeling?
(Ex. happy/sad, worried/hopeful, etc.)

_____

_____

_____

_____

_____

_____

_____

_____

_____

_____

_____

_____

_____

_____

_____

_____

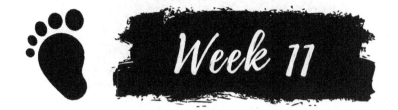

Week 11

Write about your birth or adoption story. Did it turn out how you expected?

_____

_____

_____

_____

_____

_____

_____

_____

_____

_____

_____

_____

_____

_____

_____

_____

_____

_____

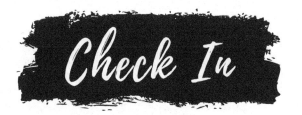

Check In

How are you feeling?

_____
_____
_____
_____
_____
_____
_____
_____
_____
_____
_____
_____
_____
_____
_____

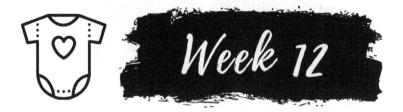

Week 12

What's your favorite thing about your baby?

_____

_____

_____

_____

_____

_____

_____

_____

_____

_____

_____

_____

_____

_____

_____

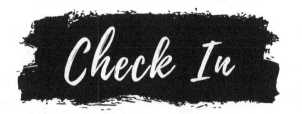

Check In

How are you feeling?

_____
_____
_____
_____
_____
_____
_____
_____
_____
_____
_____
_____
_____
_____
_____

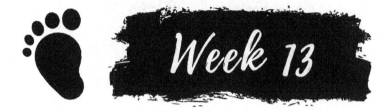

Week 13

What's your #1 worry about your baby? What can you do about it?

_____
_____
_____
_____
_____
_____
_____
_____
_____
_____
_____
_____
_____
_____
_____
_____

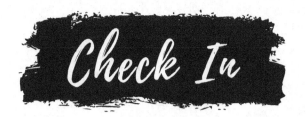

Check In

How are you feeling?

Need help? Check out the New Mommy Resources page
in the back of the book.

_____

_____

_____

_____

_____

_____

_____

_____

_____

_____

_____

_____

_____

_____

_____

_____

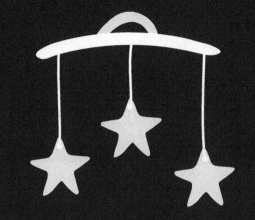

HELLO
Beautiful

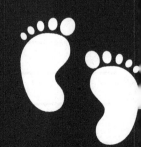

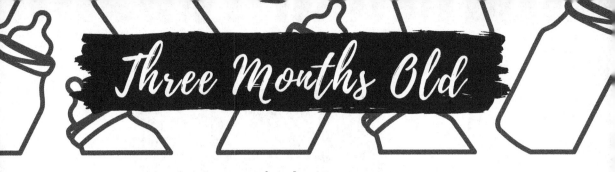

Three Months Old

My Baby's Stats
(Height, Weight, Percentiles, etc.)

_____

_____

_____

New Things My Baby Can Do

_____

_____

_____

Things My Baby Likes

_____

_____

Things My Baby Does NOT Like

_____

_____

Favorite memory or mommy accomplishment this month

_____

_____

_____

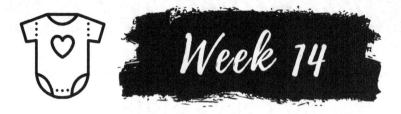

Week 14

Describe what motherhood is to you.

_____

_____

_____

_____

_____

_____

_____

_____

_____

_____

_____

_____

_____

_____

_____

_____

_____

_____

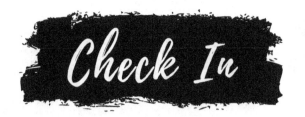

Check In

How are you feeling?
(Ex. happy/sad, worried/hopeful, etc.)

_____

_____

_____

_____

_____

_____

_____

_____

_____

_____

_____

_____

_____

_____

_____

_____

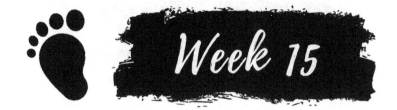

Week 15

Write about your toughest day from the past few weeks. What did you learn from it?

_____

_____

_____

_____

_____

_____

_____

_____

_____

_____

_____

_____

_____

_____

_____

_____

_____

_____

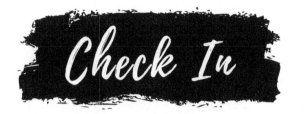

Check In

How are you feeling?

_____
_____
_____
_____
_____
_____
_____
_____
_____
_____
_____
_____
_____
_____
_____
_____
_____

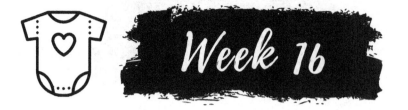

Week 16

What's something you miss from pregnancy or before?

_____
_____
_____
_____
_____
_____
_____
_____
_____
_____
_____
_____
_____
_____
_____
_____
_____
_____
_____

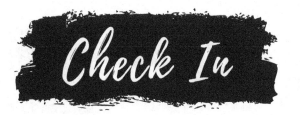

Check In

How are you feeling?

_____

_____

_____

_____

_____

_____

_____

_____

_____

_____

_____

_____

_____

_____

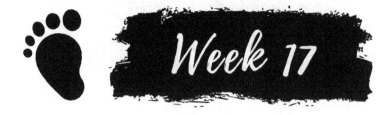

Week 17

What's the cutest thing that your baby has done?

_____

_____

_____

_____

_____

_____

_____

_____

_____

_____

_____

_____

_____

_____

_____

_____

_____

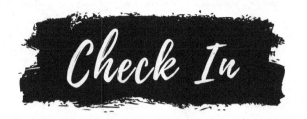

Check In

How are you feeling?
Need help? Check out the New Mommy Resources page
in the back of the book.

You
got this,
MAMA

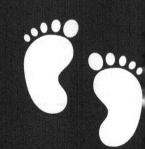

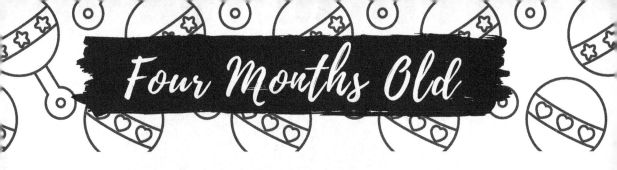

Four Months Old

My Baby's Stats
(Height, Weight, Percentiles, etc.)

_____

_____

_____

New Things My Baby Can Do

_____

_____

_____

Things My Baby Likes

_____

_____

Things My Baby Does NOT Like

_____

_____

Favorite memory or mommy accomplishment this month

_____

_____

_____

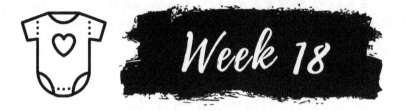

Week 18

What's the **best** advice you received about being a mom?

_____

_____

_____

_____

_____

_____

_____

_____

_____

_____

_____

_____

_____

_____

_____

_____

_____

_____

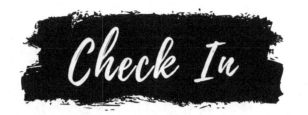

Check In

How are you feeling?
(Ex. happy/sad, worried/hopeful, etc.)

_____
_____
_____
_____
_____
_____
_____
_____
_____
_____
_____
_____
_____
_____
_____
_____

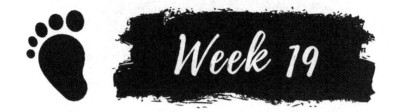

Week 19

What's the **most rewarding** part about being a mommy?

_____
_____
_____
_____
_____
_____
_____
_____
_____
_____
_____
_____
_____
_____
_____
_____

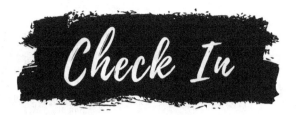

Check In

How are you feeling?

_____

_____

_____

_____

_____

_____

_____

_____

_____

_____

_____

_____

_____

_____

_____

_____

_____

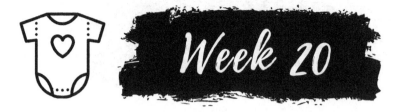

Week 20

What's one area you could give yourself a break on?

(Remember nobody is perfect.)

_____
_____
_____
_____
_____
_____
_____
_____
_____
_____
_____
_____
_____
_____
_____
_____
_____

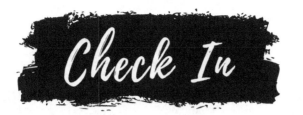

Check In

How are you feeling?

_____

_____

_____

_____

_____

_____

_____

_____

_____

_____

_____

_____

_____

_____

_____

_____

_____

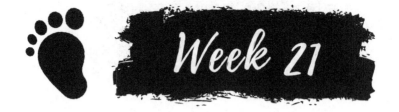

Week 21

What things are you looking forward to the most as your child grows up?

_____
_____
_____
_____
_____
_____
_____
_____
_____
_____
_____
_____
_____
_____
_____
_____
_____
_____

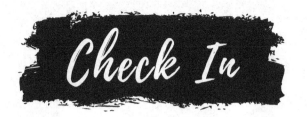

How are you feeling?

Need help? Check out the New Mommy Resources page
in the back of the book.

_____

_____

_____

_____

_____

_____

_____

_____

_____

_____

_____

_____

_____

_____

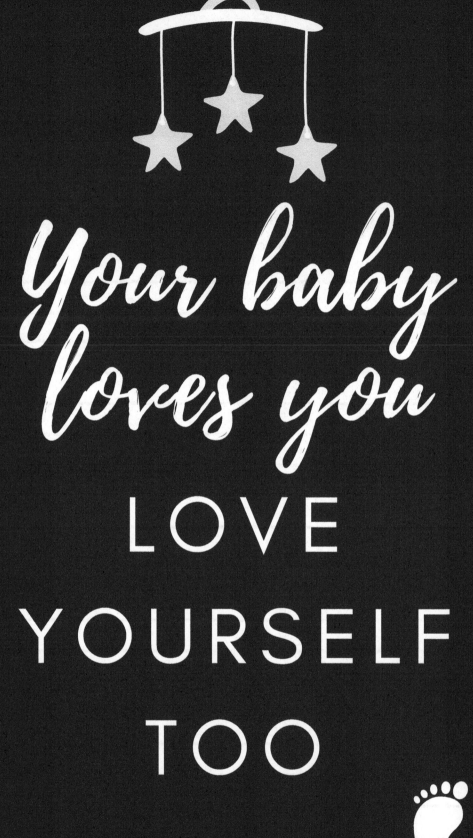

Your baby
loves you

LOVE
YOURSELF
TOO

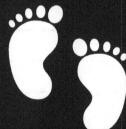

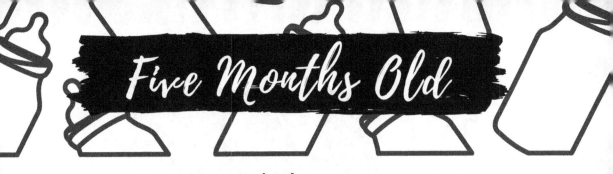

Five Months Old

My Baby's Stats
(Height, Weight, Percentiles, etc.)

_____

_____

_____

New Things My Baby Can Do

_____

_____

_____

Things My Baby Likes

_____

_____

Things My Baby Does NOT Like

_____

_____

Favorite memory or mommy accomplishment this month

_____

_____

_____

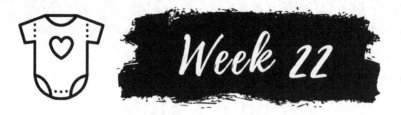

Week 22

Though their looks seem to change every day, who does your child look like?

_____

_____

_____

_____

_____

_____

_____

_____

_____

_____

_____

_____

_____

_____

_____

_____

_____

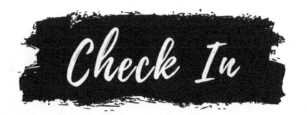

Check In

How are you feeling?
(Ex. happy/sad, worried/hopeful, etc.)

_____
_____
_____
_____
_____
_____
_____
_____
_____
_____
_____
_____
_____
_____
_____
_____

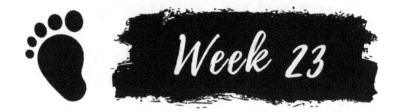

Week 23

Congratulations, you made it to the six month mark! Now that your baby is older, what changes do you see?

_____

_____

_____

_____

_____

_____

_____

_____

_____

_____

_____

_____

_____

_____

_____

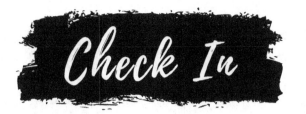

Check In

How are you feeling?

_____
_____
_____
_____
_____
_____
_____
_____
_____
_____
_____
_____
_____
_____
_____
_____

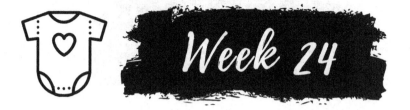

Week 24

Does your baby's name and
personality match? Why or why not?

_____

_____

_____

_____

_____

_____

_____

_____

_____

_____

_____

_____

_____

_____

_____

_____

_____

_____

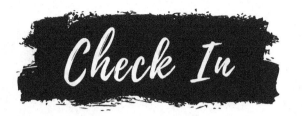

Check In

How are you feeling?

_____
_____
_____
_____
_____
_____
_____
_____
_____
_____
_____
_____
_____
_____

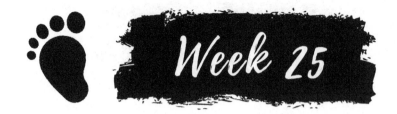

Week 25

How have you changed since becoming a mom?

_____

_____

_____

_____

_____

_____

_____

_____

_____

_____

_____

_____

_____

_____

_____

_____

_____

_____

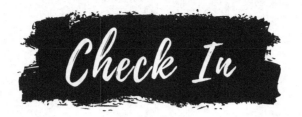

Check In

How are you feeling?
Need help? Check out the New Mommy Resources page in the back of the book.

_____

_____

_____

_____

_____

_____

_____

_____

_____

_____

_____

_____

_____

_____

_____

_____

_____

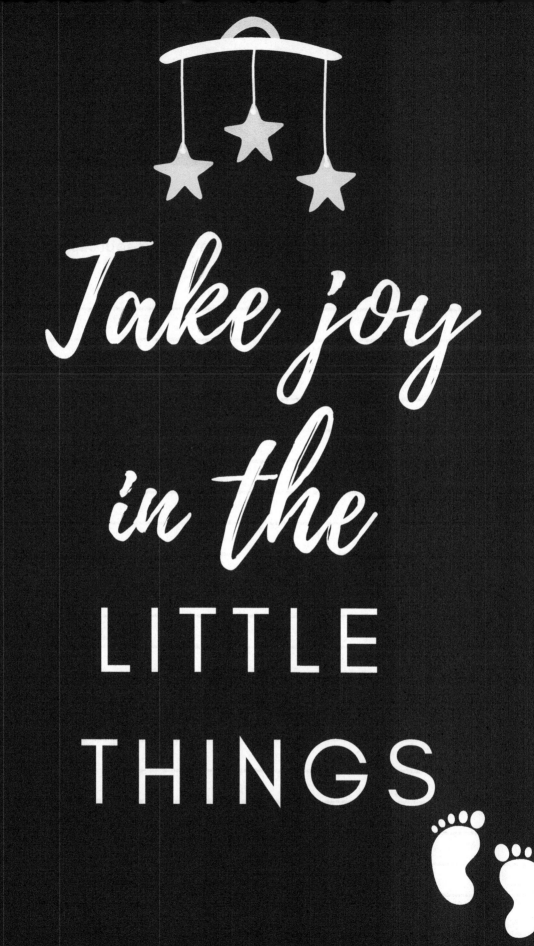

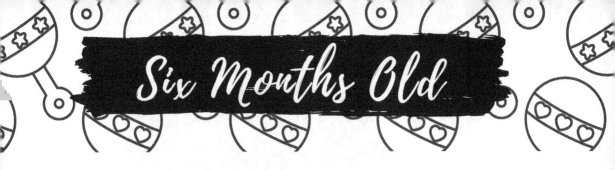

Six Months Old

My Baby's Stats
(Height, Weight, Percentiles, etc.)

_____

_____

_____

New Things My Baby Can Do

_____

_____

_____

Things My Baby Likes

_____

_____

Things My Baby Does NOT Like

_____

_____

Favorite memory or mommy accomplishment this month

_____

_____

_____

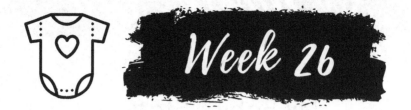

Week 26

What's one thing you wish someone would have told you about being a mom?

_____

_____

_____

_____

_____

_____

_____

_____

_____

_____

_____

_____

_____

_____

_____

_____

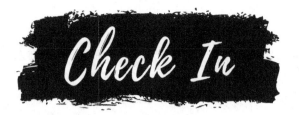

Check In

How are you feeling?
(Ex. happy/sad, worried/hopeful, etc.)

_____
_____
_____
_____
_____
_____
_____
_____
_____
_____
_____
_____
_____
_____
_____
_____
_____
_____

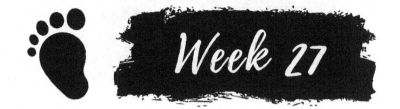

Week 27

Write down a thought you've never
said out loud. How did writing about
it make you feel?

_____
_____
_____
_____
_____
_____
_____
_____
_____
_____
_____
_____
_____
_____
_____
_____

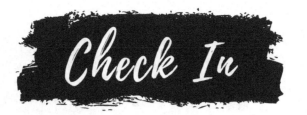

Check In

How are you feeling?

_____
_____
_____
_____
_____
_____
_____
_____
_____
_____
_____
_____
_____
_____
_____

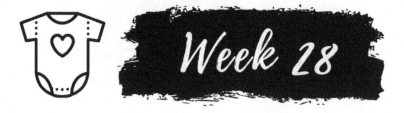

Week 28

Share a dream you have about your child's future.

_____
_____
_____
_____
_____
_____
_____
_____
_____
_____
_____
_____
_____
_____
_____
_____
_____
_____

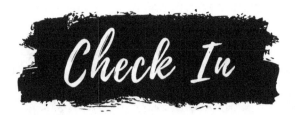

Check In

How are you feeling?

_____
_____
_____
_____
_____
_____
_____
_____
_____
_____
_____
_____
_____
_____
_____
_____

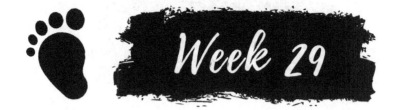

Week 29

How can your spouse/family/friends help you? After you write, be sure to share with them.

_____
_____
_____
_____
_____
_____
_____
_____
_____
_____
_____
_____
_____
_____
_____
_____

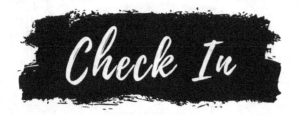

Check In

How are you feeling?

Need help? Check out the New Mommy Resources page
in the back of the book.

_____

_____

_____

_____

_____

_____

_____

_____

_____

_____

_____

_____

_____

_____

_____

_____

_____

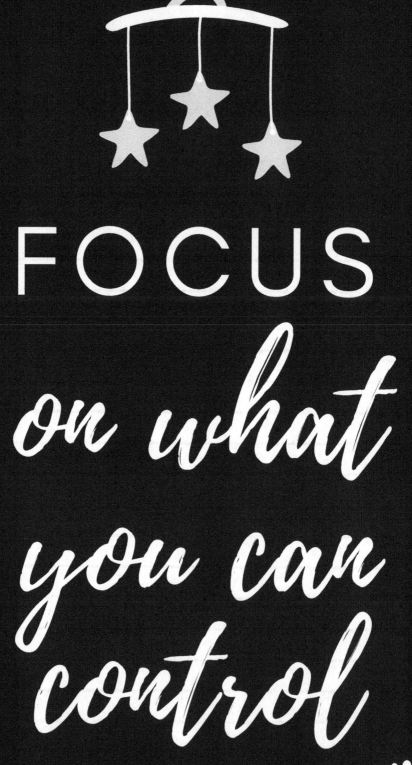

FOCUS

on what you can control

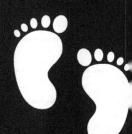

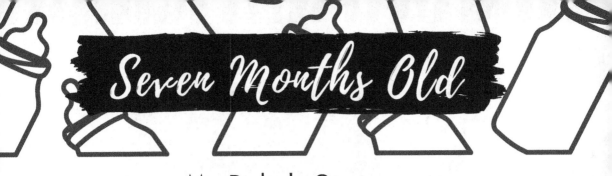

Seven Months Old

My Baby's Stats
(Height, Weight, Percentiles, etc.)

_____

_____

_____

New Things My Baby Can Do

_____

_____

_____

Things My Baby Likes

_____

_____

Things My Baby Does NOT Like

_____

_____

Favorite memory or mommy accomplishment this month

_____

_____

_____

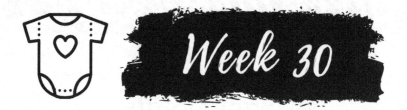

Week 30

What struggles or worries do/did you have with feeding your baby?

(Remember to get help on the resources page.)

_____
_____
_____
_____
_____
_____
_____
_____
_____
_____
_____
_____
_____
_____
_____
_____

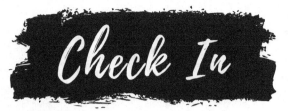

Check In

How are you feeling?
(Ex. happy/sad, worried/hopeful, etc.)

_____

_____

_____

_____

_____

_____

_____

_____

_____

_____

_____

_____

_____

_____

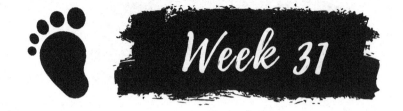

Week 31

What steps can/did you take to start feeling like yourself again?

_____

_____

_____

_____

_____

_____

_____

_____

_____

_____

_____

_____

_____

_____

_____

_____

_____

_____

_____

_____

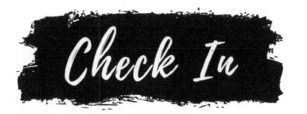

Check In

How are you feeling?

_____
_____
_____
_____
_____
_____
_____
_____
_____
_____
_____
_____
_____
_____
_____
_____
_____

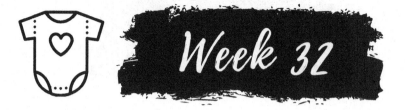

Week 32

Describe how you felt when your baby
first recognized your voice or face.

_____
_____
_____
_____
_____
_____
_____
_____
_____
_____
_____
_____
_____
_____
_____

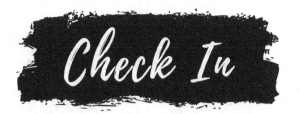

How are you feeling?

_____

_____

_____

_____

_____

_____

_____

_____

_____

_____

_____

_____

_____

_____

_____

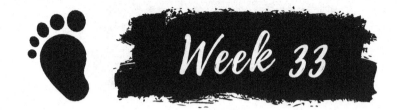

Week 33

How has your relationship with your partner/spouse changed since having your child?

_____

_____

_____

_____

_____

_____

_____

_____

_____

_____

_____

_____

_____

_____

_____

_____

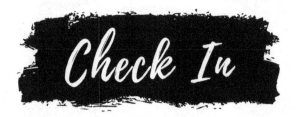

Check In

How are you feeling?

Need help? Check out the New Mommy Resources page
in the back of the book.

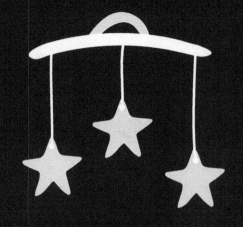

Stay
STRONG

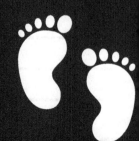

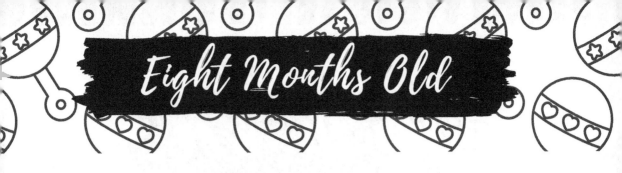

Eight Months Old

My Baby's Stats
(Height, Weight, Percentiles, etc.)

_____

_____

_____

New Things My Baby Can Do

_____

_____

_____

Things My Baby Likes

_____

_____

Things My Baby Does NOT Like

_____

_____

Favorite memory or mommy accomplishment this month

_____

_____

_____

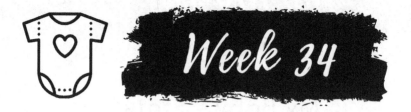

Week 34

Write about the time you first saw
your baby smile.

_____
_____
_____
_____
_____
_____
_____
_____
_____
_____
_____
_____
_____
_____
_____
_____
_____

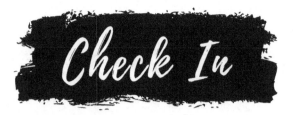

Check In

How are you feeling?
(Ex. happy/sad, worried/hopeful, etc.)

_____
_____
_____
_____
_____
_____
_____
_____
_____
_____
_____
_____
_____
_____
_____
_____
_____

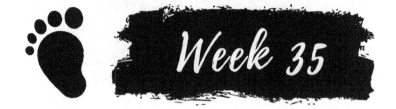

Week 35

When did you start to feel the most connected to your baby?

_____
_____
_____
_____
_____
_____
_____
_____
_____
_____
_____
_____
_____
_____
_____
_____
_____
_____

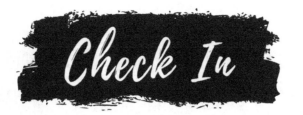

Check In

How are you feeling?

_____
_____
_____
_____
_____
_____
_____
_____
_____
_____
_____
_____
_____
_____
_____
_____

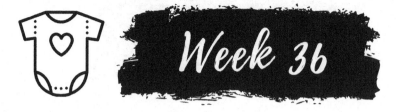

Week 36

What's the **hardest** part about being a mother?

_____
_____
_____
_____
_____
_____
_____
_____
_____
_____
_____
_____
_____
_____
_____
_____
_____

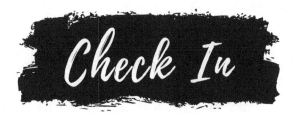

Check In

How are you feeling?

_____
_____
_____
_____
_____
_____
_____
_____
_____
_____
_____
_____
_____
_____
_____
_____
_____
_____
_____

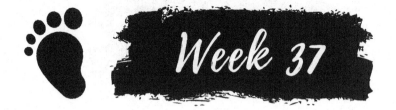

Week 37

Are you the mother you thought you would be? Why or why not?

_____
_____
_____
_____
_____
_____
_____
_____
_____
_____
_____
_____
_____
_____
_____
_____
_____
_____
_____

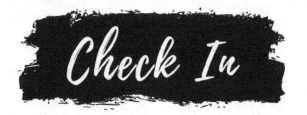

Check In

How are you feeling?

Need help? Check out the New Mommy Resources page
in the back of the book.

_____

_____

_____

_____

_____

_____

_____

_____

_____

_____

_____

_____

_____

_____

_____

_____

_____

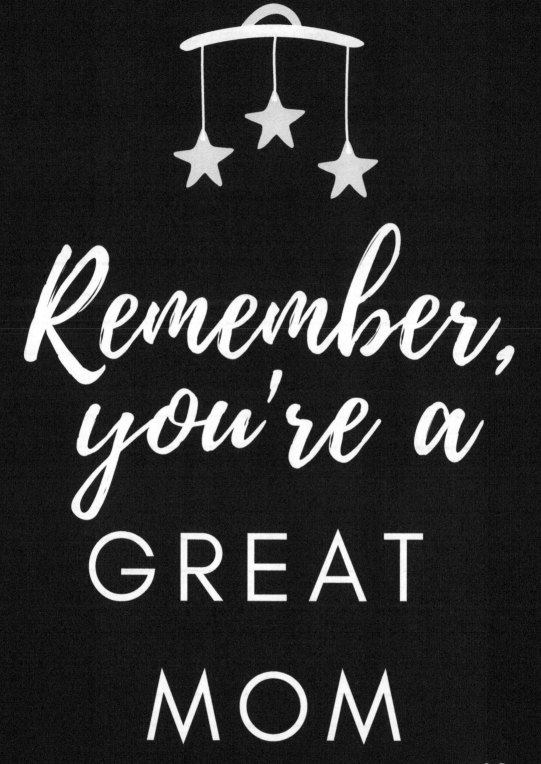

Remember, you're a GREAT MOM

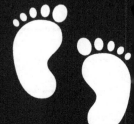

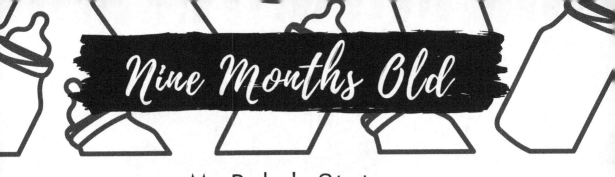

Nine Months Old

My Baby's Stats
(Height, Weight, Percentiles, etc.)

_____

_____

_____

New Things My Baby Can Do

_____

_____

_____

Things My Baby Likes

_____

_____

Things My Baby Does NOT Like

_____

_____

Favorite memory or mommy accomplishment this month

_____

_____

_____

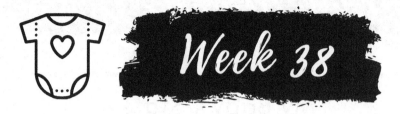

Week 38

What made you start to feel like a mom?

_____
_____
_____
_____
_____
_____
_____
_____
_____
_____
_____
_____
_____
_____
_____
_____
_____

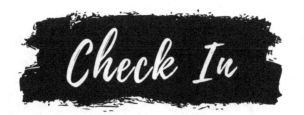

Check In

How are you feeling?
(Ex. happy/sad, worried/hopeful, etc.)

_____
_____
_____
_____
_____
_____
_____
_____
_____
_____
_____
_____
_____
_____

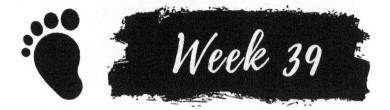

Week 39

Where's the first place you took your baby? How did you feel?

(No, the doctor's office doesn't count!)

_____

_____

_____

_____

_____

_____

_____

_____

_____

_____

_____

_____

_____

_____

_____

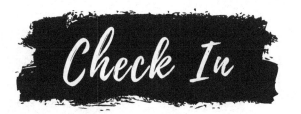

Check In

How are you feeling?

_____
_____
_____
_____
_____
_____
_____
_____
_____
_____
_____
_____
_____
_____
_____
_____
_____

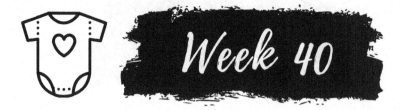

Week 40

What kind of mom pressure are you feeling or criticism are you facing?

_____
_____
_____
_____
_____
_____
_____
_____
_____
_____
_____
_____
_____
_____
_____
_____
_____
_____
_____

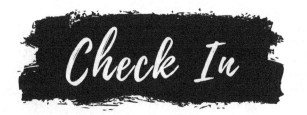

How are you feeling?

_____

_____

_____

_____

_____

_____

_____

_____

_____

_____

_____

_____

_____

_____

_____

_____

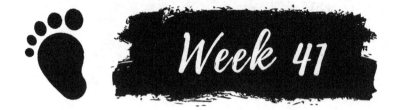

Week 41

What's one thing you used to worry about that you now don't anymore?

_____
_____
_____
_____
_____
_____
_____
_____
_____
_____
_____
_____
_____
_____
_____
_____
_____
_____
_____

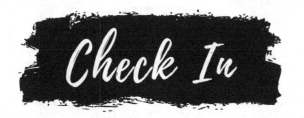

Check In

How are you feeling?

Need help? Check out the New Mommy Resources page
in the back of the book.

_____

_____

_____

_____

_____

_____

_____

_____

_____

_____

_____

_____

_____

_____

_____

_____

_____

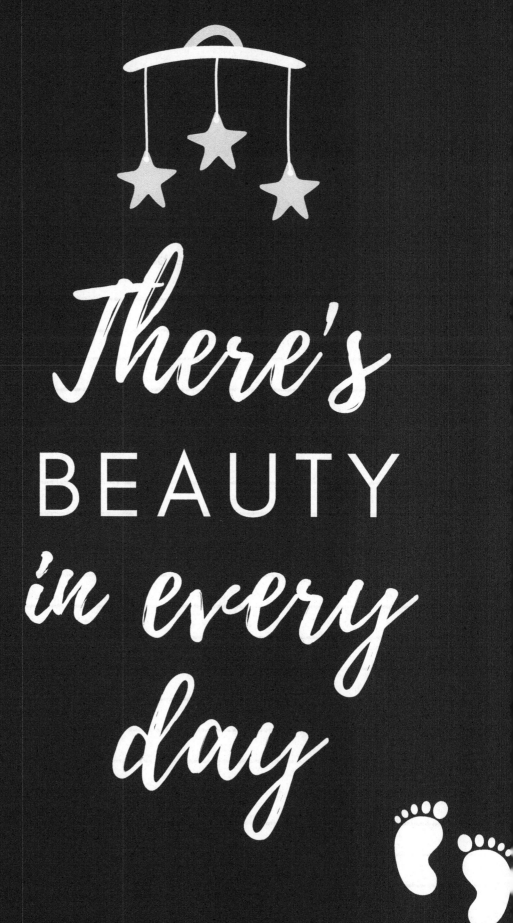

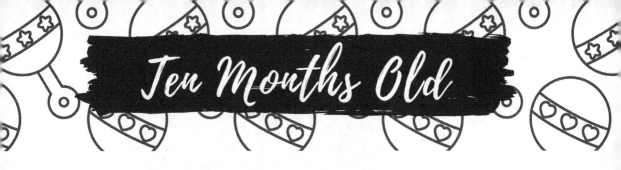

Ten Months Old

My Baby's Stats
(Height, Weight, Percentiles, etc.)

_____

_____

_____

New Things My Baby Can Do

_____

_____

_____

Things My Baby Likes

_____

_____

Things My Baby Does NOT Like

_____

_____

Favorite memory or mommy accomplishment this month

_____

_____

_____

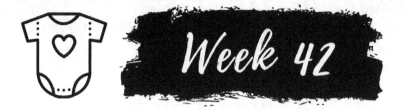

Week 42

How can you take care of yourself today?

(Go for a walk, eat a treat, take a bath, etc.)

_____

_____

_____

_____

_____

_____

_____

_____

_____

_____

_____

_____

_____

_____

_____

_____

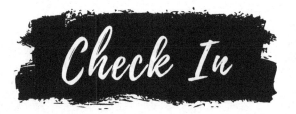

Check In

How are you feeling?
(Ex. happy/sad, worried/hopeful, etc.)

_____
_____
_____
_____
_____
_____
_____
_____
_____
_____
_____
_____
_____
_____
_____
_____

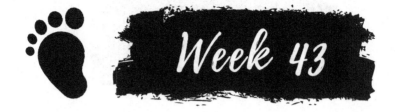

Week 43

What's your favorite part of being a mommy?

_____
_____
_____
_____
_____
_____
_____
_____
_____
_____
_____
_____
_____
_____
_____
_____
_____

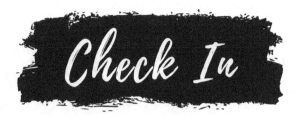

Check In

How are you feeling?

_____

_____

_____

_____

_____

_____

_____

_____

_____

_____

_____

_____

_____

_____

_____

_____

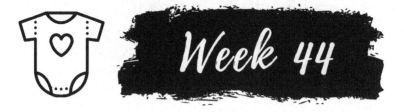

Week 44

What's one thing you'd change about your motherhood journey?

_____
_____
_____
_____
_____
_____
_____
_____
_____
_____
_____
_____
_____
_____
_____
_____
_____

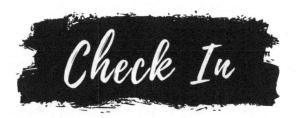

Check In

How are you feeling?

_____
_____
_____
_____
_____
_____
_____
_____
_____
_____
_____
_____
_____
_____
_____
_____
_____

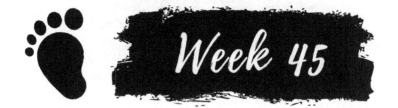

Week 45

Make a list of some moms you can connect with, and write what you want to talk about or ask them.

_____
_____
_____
_____
_____
_____
_____
_____
_____
_____
_____
_____
_____
_____
_____
_____
_____

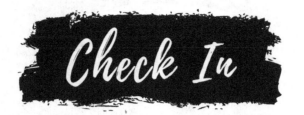

Check In

How are you feeling?

Need help? Check out the New Mommy Resources page
in the back of the book.

_____

_____

_____

_____

_____

_____

_____

_____

_____

_____

_____

_____

_____

_____

_____

_____

_____

_____

Just
BREATHE

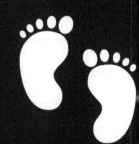

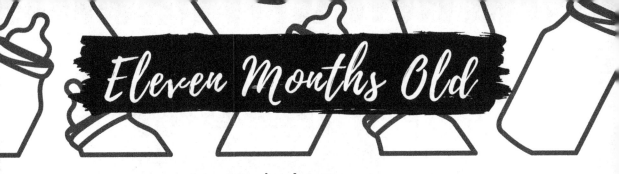

Eleven Months Old

My Baby's Stats
(Height, Weight, Percentiles, etc.)

_____

_____

_____

New Things My Baby Can Do

_____

_____

_____

Things My Baby Likes

_____

_____

Things My Baby Does NOT Like

_____

_____

Favorite memory or mommy accomplishment this month

_____

_____

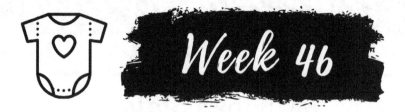

Week 46

What do you REALLY think about your post baby body? Be honest.

_____

_____

_____

_____

_____

_____

_____

_____

_____

_____

_____

_____

_____

_____

_____

_____

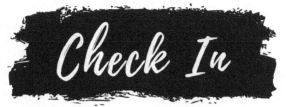

Check In

How are you feeling?
(Ex. happy/sad, worried/hopeful, etc.)

_____

_____

_____

_____

_____

_____

_____

_____

_____

_____

_____

_____

_____

_____

_____

_____

_____

_____

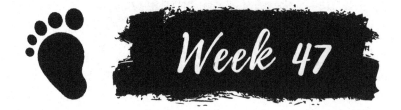

Week 47

What's been the biggest transition to life with a baby?

_____
_____
_____
_____
_____
_____
_____
_____
_____
_____
_____
_____
_____
_____
_____
_____
_____

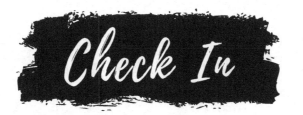

Check In

How are you feeling?

_____
_____
_____
_____
_____
_____
_____
_____
_____
_____
_____
_____
_____
_____
_____
_____

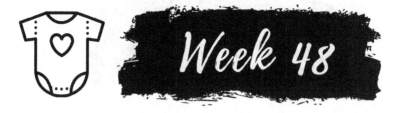

Week 48

How has your mothering changed over the past year?

_____
_____
_____
_____
_____
_____
_____
_____
_____
_____
_____
_____
_____
_____
_____
_____

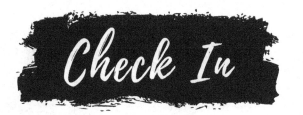

Check In

How are you feeling?

_____

_____

_____

_____

_____

_____

_____

_____

_____

_____

_____

_____

_____

_____

_____

_____

_____

_____

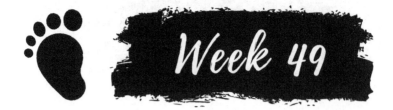

Week 49

What's one way that you're stronger than you were before?

_____
_____
_____
_____
_____
_____
_____
_____
_____
_____
_____
_____
_____
_____
_____
_____
_____
_____

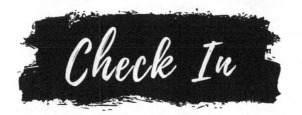

Check In

How are you feeling?
Need help? Check out the New Mommy Resources page
in the back of the book.

_____

_____

_____

_____

_____

_____

_____

_____

_____

_____

_____

_____

_____

_____

_____

_____

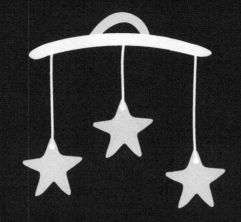

SOAK UP

the sweet

memories

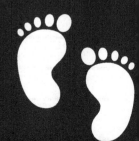

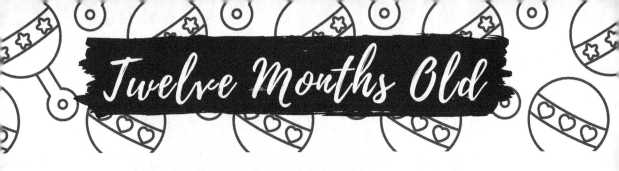

Twelve Months Old

My Baby's Stats
(Height, Weight, Percentiles, etc.)

_____

_____

_____

New Things My Baby Can Do

_____

_____

_____

Things My Baby Likes

_____

_____

Things My Baby Does NOT Like

_____

_____

Favorite memory or mommy accomplishment this month

_____

_____

_____

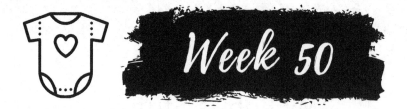

Week 50

What's one thing you won't miss from this first year?

_____
_____
_____
_____
_____
_____
_____
_____
_____
_____
_____
_____
_____
_____
_____
_____
_____
_____

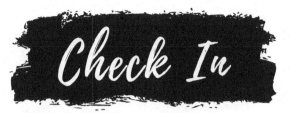

Check In

How are you feeling?
(Ex. happy/sad, worried/hopeful, etc.)

_____

_____

_____

_____

_____

_____

_____

_____

_____

_____

_____

_____

_____

_____

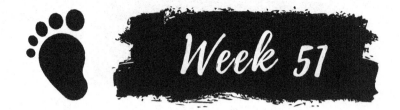

Week 51

How has your relationship with or feelings about your mother changed since becoming a mom?

_____

_____

_____

_____

_____

_____

_____

_____

_____

_____

_____

_____

_____

_____

_____

_____

_____

_____

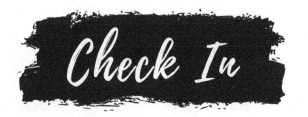

Check In

How are you feeling?

_____

_____

_____

_____

_____

_____

_____

_____

_____

_____

_____

_____

_____

_____

_____

_____

_____

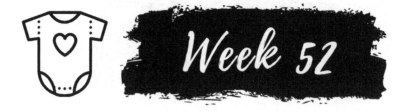

Week 52

Your baby is officially no longer a
baby. How does that make you feel?

_____
_____
_____
_____
_____
_____
_____
_____
_____
_____
_____
_____
_____
_____
_____
_____
_____

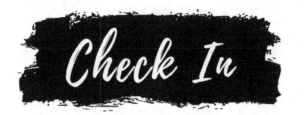

Check In

How are you feeling?

Need help? Check out the New Mommy Resources page
in the back of the book.

_____

_____

_____

_____

_____

_____

_____

_____

_____

_____

_____

_____

_____

_____

_____

_____

_____

_____

_____

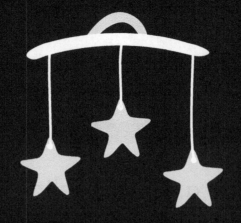

CELEBRATE

each and every win

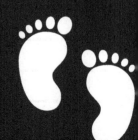

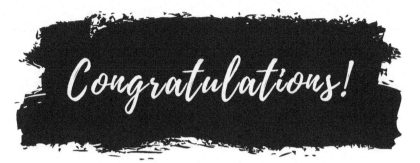

Congratulations!

You survived your first year! Reflect on how your life has changed in the past 12 months.

_____

_____

_____

_____

_____

_____

_____

_____

_____

_____

_____

_____

_____

_____

_____

_____

_____

Notes

Here's a place for all those extra thoughts that might pop into your head.

Notes

Here's a place for all those extra thoughts that might pop into your head.

Notes

Here's a place for all those extra thoughts that might pop into your head.

Notes

Here's a place for all those extra thoughts that might pop into your head.

Notes

Here's a place for all those extra thoughts that might pop into your head.

Notes

Here's a place for all those extra
thoughts that might pop into your head.

Mommy Resources

Visit www.ChefAshleyShep.com/newmom for resources to support you on this new mom journey. There you'll find help with baby blues, breastfeeding, and more. You'll also find recipes, tips, and strategies to get dinner done faster. Who wants to spend all day in the kitchen when you could be enjoying baby snuggles? Since you're probably too tired to type the website in, just use the directions below to be taken directly to the site.

If you're feeling overwhelmed, stressed, or anxious, then it might be time to talk to your doctor and/or a therapist. It's totally normal to feel this way, but know that you don't have to stay that way. Remember to reach out if you need to, even if it's just a text to a fellow mommy friend. At times, I felt guilty about having baby blues. My son was an angel, and I didn't have any "real" complications with my pregnancy or labor. It was still important to acknowledge my feelings to be able to work through them. Make sure you do the same for you. Check out the resources found at www.ChefAshleyShep.com/newmom or scan the QR code below.

Open the camera app on your smartphone and place it over the image below to be taken to quick, healthy recipes as well as new mom tips. Remember to reach out to someone if you need to if you're not feeling like yourself.

About the Author

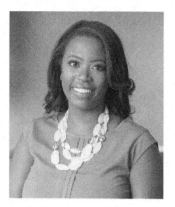

Ashley D. Shepard is a wife, mom, personal chef, and mealtime strategist (also known as Chef Ashley Shep). She helps busy moms get dinner done faster with quick, healthy meals that taste good.

Visit www.ChefAshleyShep.com/newmom (or scan the QR code below) to find easy ways to feed your family as well new mom resources to help you on this journey.

You can follow her @ChefAshleyShep on Facebook, Instagram, Pinterest, and YouTube. To get started, open the camera app on your smartphone and place it over the image below to be taken to quick, healthy recipes as well as new mom resources.

Made in the USA
Monee, IL
16 December 2021

85952593R00085